LOSE BELLY FAT

A Blueprint to Fit Into Those Jeans!

Jo Hansen

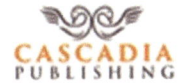

CASCADIA
PUBLISHING

www.cascadiapublishing.com

Legal & Disclaimer

The information contained in this book and its contents is not designed to replace or take the place of any form of medical or professional advice; and is not meant to replace the need for independent medical, financial, legal or other professional advice or services, as may be required. The content and information in this book has been provided for educational and entertainment purposes only.

The content and information contained in this book has been compiled from sources deemed reliable, and it is accurate to the best of the Author's knowledge, information and belief. However, the Author cannot guarantee its accuracy and validity and cannot be held liable for any errors and/or omissions. Further, changes are periodically made to this book as and when needed. Where appropriate and/or necessary, you must consult a professional (including but not limited to your doctor, attorney, financial advisor or such other professional advisor) before using any of the suggested remedies, techniques, or information in this book.

Upon using the contents and information contained in this book, you agree to hold harmless the Author from and against any damages, costs, and expenses, including any legal fees potentially resulting from the application of any of the information provided by this book. This disclaimer applies to any loss, damages or injury caused by the use and application, whether directly or indirectly, of any advice or information presented, whether for breach of contract, tort, negligence, personal injury, criminal intent, or under any other cause of action.

You agree to accept all risks of using the information presented inside this book.

You agree that by continuing to read this book, where appropriate and/or necessary, you shall consult a professional (including but not limited to your doctor, attorney, or financial advisor or such other advisor as needed) before using any of the suggested remedies, techniques, or information in this book.

Table of Contents

Introduction

No one wants to have belly fat. Aside from being unsightly, having excess fats in your belly can also hamper your health and lower your stamina. According to research, fat is crucial for survival, but only the healthy type and if taken in moderation. Healthy fats can provide your body with energy, especially if you were not able to consume foods that are supposed to provide you with the amount of energy that you need.

The ability of fat to provide energy is one of the reasons why people during the past ate processed and fat-rich foods, especially when there is food shortage. This allowed them to survive because these foods were able to sustain their energy for a long time. However, eating too much processed and fat-rich foods is no longer applicable during the modern times. It is because the lifestyle of most people now is more sedentary than in the past.

Everything is also fast-paced, and with the advanced technology that we have right now, physical movements that are essential in burning the excess fats that we consume are already hard to accomplish. The increasing number of fast food chains and overly processed foods also contribute to some people's unhealthy and sedentary lifestyle. With that in mind, it is no longer surprising to see obesity as one of the most common issues affecting developed countries like Japan, US, and other European countries.

The irony is that it is harder to reduce fat than gain it; this is the main reason why there are numerous attempts to help modern people aiming to get rid of their excessive fat. This gives rise to several diet plans, weight loss supplements and workout programs.

If you are one of those who wish to get rid of stubborn fats, especially in the belly, then this book is for you. It will serve as an extensive guide to lose belly fat fast. Note that the belly is where most fats are stored. When you gain weight, the excess fats will most likely fill the inner layer of your belly first then move to the lower parts of your body like the hips, thighs and bottoms. The upper parts of the body, including the cheeks, neck, shoulders and arms, are where the excess fats will most likely accumulate last.

If you don't get rid of these excess fats properly, then there is a great possibility that these will damage your internal organs, causing you to experience plenty of health issues. Accumulating too much fats will also cause your internal organs to store them. To avoid ruining your overall health, you need to get rid of them.

The good news is that it is now possible to get rid of excess belly fats through proper diet and the right exercises. You are on the right path when you purchase this book. It contains numerous fat burning exercises plus a 2-week diet plan so you can finally let go of your unhealthy habits and replace them with healthy ones. You will also find a lot of useful strategies in maintaining your flat belly forever through this book. Be ready to reveal a newer and healthier you and flaunt a slimmer body and flatter stomach after reading this book and following through each of the strategies mentioned here.

Happy reading!

Chapter 1 - Where All the Fat Come?

Excessive belly fat has many causes – one of which is your unhealthy food choices and another is your inactive or sedentary lifestyle. Hormonal imbalance can also trigger the unwanted storage of fats in your belly. With the many causes of unwanted belly fats, it is just right to dedicate a chapter to discuss most, if not all of them. By identifying their actual causes, finding the most suitable solutions to minimize or get rid of them will be easier. Here are just some of these causes:

1. Unhealthy Food Choices

Excessive consumption of unhealthy foods, particularly those with high levels of sugar, can cause most parts of your body, especially the belly to accumulate fats. The way you consume foods can actually be attributed to the habits that you have developed throughout the years. This means that if you are used to eating too much foods all at once or eating two meals with just a very short gap in between, then it is greatly possible for your body to accumulate too much calories and fats from them, causing it to be unable to use all the energy it produces.

Your unhealthy food choices can also hamper your metabolism. The intake of too much calorie- and fat-laden foods may cause almost all parts of your body, especially the belly to store more fats. This is the main reason why a lot of experts advise those who wish to lose weight to reduce their food consumption. If possible, eat only whenever you feel hungry and make sure to stop eating before you feel full. Remember that your body normally needs up to 20 minutes to recognize that it is already full, so please stop eating even if you don't feel full yet.

It is also advisable to lengthen the gap between two big meals. Avoid eating too often. While it is okay to grab snacks during that gap, make sure to choose the healthy kinds – ex. fruits and veggies. Avoid consuming foods that are rich in starch, carbs and sugars as these can only cause you to gain more weight. Your diet should also consist of healthy foods.

2. Nervousness and Other Negative Emotions

Your current mental condition also plays a major role in your metabolism. For instance, if you feel depressed due to overwhelming stress, anxiety and pressures, then there is a great possibility that you will experience hunger. It is mainly because your body will crave for foods, especially sugary ones that can make you feel calmer and happier. If you are suffering from stress, then it is most likely that your cravings for sweets like chocolates and candies will intensify. You will also most likely crave for more coffee, tea and alcoholic beverages.

All these foods and drinks have high amounts of sugar that, when stored in your body, may develop into fat. If your weight gain is mainly caused by stress, nervousness or other negative emotions, then the first step to solving it is to handle the negative emotion first. Improve your mental and psychological condition. Note that no matter how hard you diet or exercise, you won't get your desired results if you don't solve the main problem. Try to make yourself feel better emotionally before starting any diet or workout regimen.

3. Hormonal Imbalance

This usually affects those who are already between 30 and 50. Hormonal changes or imbalance most likely happen to women during their menstrual cycle, pregnancy or menopausal stage. Unhealthy working habits can also trigger an imbalance in your hormones. Increasing the number of your physical activities is one of the main solutions to addressing this kind of problem. Avoid spending too much idle time, or sitting in front of your computer for too long. Perform some workouts that will reduce belly fats and correct your hormonal imbalance.

4. Excessive Alcohol Intake

Excessive alcohol intake may also cause you to accumulate fats in your belly, which others call as beer belly. Since the main trigger is alcohol, you need to reduce or fully eliminate it from your diet. You also need to stay away from other beverages with high sugar content, like soft drinks or carbonated drinks and packaged juice, since these also stimulate the development of belly fats.

5. Genetics

Some people say that if obesity is genetically inherited from your parents or ancestors, you cannot do much about it. This myth is entirely wrong. Even if your case is hereditary or due to genetics, it is still possible to resolve it with the right workout and diet plan. You can do workouts regularly like running, walking, hiking or climbing stairs, and eat healthy foods to ensure that you can maintain a slimmer body and flatter belly.

6. Lack of Exercise

Physical activities are extremely important if you want to maintain a slim figure. If you have been active in the past then stopped all of a sudden, then you may start to develop belly fat and gain weight. If that's the case, then performing regular exercises is crucial for you. You should also eat healthy foods, and pair them with regular exercises to speed up your metabolism. Stay away from carbs, gluten, sugar, fats and starch.

To sum up everything that this chapter discussed, here are some of the most common causes of belly fat:

- Consumption of too much fat, starch, carbohydrates, gluten and sugar

- Too much alcohol, carb beverages and packaged juice intake

- Prolonged sitting

- Inadequate sleep or too much sleep within the day

- Inactivity (not having enough exercises)

- Hormonal imbalance, especially for women - menstruation, pregnancy and menopause

- Stress, anxiety, depression, and other mental and emotional problems

- Eating in big portions (excessive food intake)

By understanding the causes, you will know exactly where your belly fats come from. This is helpful in taking the right actions in reducing or fully eliminating them and preventing them from coming back.

Chapter 2 - Say NO to Instant Fat Burning Methods

I understand how hard it is for many to start a diet, stick to it and develop a healthier habit. This especially holds true if they are used to eating unhealthy foods and following unhealthy habits. This is the main reason why the weight loss industry is now filled with numerous solutions to stubborn belly fat that claim to get rid of the problem instantly. Note, however, that these instant solutions have negative consequences or side effects.

While you won't notice the effects right away, you will eventually feel them in the long run. It may take months, or even years, to see the negative effects of these instant solutions, and these can range from minor problems such as nausea and headache, to more serious and severe ones, such as cancer, heart attack, kidney failure and liver problems. This chapter will talk about some of these instant dieting solutions, as well as their individual consequences.

Liposuction

Liposuction is one of the most popular fat reduction methods with instant results. Although it costs a great amount of money, many people, especially those who can afford it, prefer to undergo the procedure to obtain a flatter stomach and a thinner body. It produces fast results, in that you visit the clinic with excess fats around your belly and in other parts of your body, and come out as a slimmer person after the procedure. However, take note that it also comes with serious health consequences including the following:

- **Fat embolism** – This condition is characterized by the loosened fats moving to your blood vessels, then transported to your brain or heart. It is severe that it can trigger further complications to your health, or can even cause death.

- **Seroma** – This condition is characterized by the formation of fluids beneath your skin, causing your skin to be bumpy. To cure this problem, you may need to undergo a painful medical procedure, which involves the removal of fluid.

- **Loose skin** – Since liposuction drains excess fats in the treated area, there is a great tendency for your skin to become loose and unattractive. In worse cases, liposuction may cause the death of the skin cells in the treated area, causing it to become darker than the rest of your body.

- **Infection** – Liposuction is a surgical procedure, which is one of the reasons why you are prone to infection when you try it out. Note that there will be open wounds from the surgery, which increases your risk of getting infection. Without proper treatment, the infection may trigger more serious health issues.

- **Inner organs failure** – Liposuction may also cause the level of fluids in your body to change dramatically, triggering fatal heart and liver problems.

- **Death** - There are several cases of death that were reported due to liposuction since its success is fully dependent on a patient's present health condition, as well as his/her ability to tolerate the procedure and its negative effects. There is no hundred percent guarantee that the procedure will be successful.

Diet Pills

Many companies nowadays offer various kinds of diet pills that claim to be effective in reducing belly fat. While some are made of herbs, making their manufacturers claim that these products are safe, natural and don't come with any side effects, you are still not one hundred percent guaranteed that these are harmless. The problem with most of these diet pills is that their negative side effects are not noticeable right away. It is mainly because the effects usually target your inner organs like your kidneys, liver and your heart.

In the United States, many diet pills were already banned, recalled, or withdrawn from the market because they contain ingredients that are harmful to the body. There were even reports of dead victims from these diet pills, as well as those who need liver or kidney transplant.

Here are some harmful effects of diet pills:

- Sleeplessness - It is because some diet pills are made of ingredients that can increase your heart rate instantly.

- High blood pressure

- Diarrhoea – This especially holds true for those who are sensitive to some of the ingredients used in the pills.

- Anxiety – Some reports show that those who take diet pills feel uncomfortable with their own bodies. Some of the pills can also cause users to become anxious and unwell.

- Increased risk of suffering from stroke and heart attack

- Kidney and liver problems – The main reason is that the pills tend to force the inner organs to work harder.

- Rectal bleeding – This usually happens once the pills start to harm your inner organs. Some pills are damaging to the colon, causing the anus to bleed.

Diet Food or Drink

Several diet foods and drinks are also available in the market. Several false advertisements continue to deceive viewers and customers with their claims that the foods and beverages that they offer are the best in the market when it comes to dieting. A wise tip is to avoid trusting any diet labels placed on these products. The main reason is that these instant diet foods and drinks also contain artificial sugars, preservatives and other chemicals, making them unhealthy. While you may not feel their effects directly, they still cause your body to accumulate more unnatural and unhealthy substances that may lead to severe health conditions or cancer in the long run.

Extreme Dieting

Extreme dieting methods have also become popular especially for those who would like to lose weight rapidly. These methods require you to force yourself to do something extreme just to reach your target weight at your target date. One example of extreme dieting method is forcing yourself to eliminate salt from your diet for a specific duration. Another is getting rid of carbs from your diet completely and substituting it with more portions of healthy fats and protein. If left unmanaged, the mentioned dieting methods can cause several problems including the following:

- **Excessive fatigue** – It is because your body will most likely get weak and exhausted from the entire procedure.

- **Nausea** – The extreme dieting method can cause utmost discomfort within your body, causing you to experience vomiting and nausea.

- **Mineral / nutritional deficiency** – This will happen if you force yourself to get rid of a certain nutrient or mineral from your diet, such as salt, just to reach your target weight.

- **Increased cholesterol level** - Imbalanced diet - such as consuming too much fat with the hope that it will be processed into energy – has adverse side effects including increased cholesterol level and high blood pressure.

Extreme Fat Burning Exercises

Taking too much time in the gym or over-exercising is also not a good idea. Avoid thinking that the more workouts you do and the more time you spend in the gym exercising, the healthier and slimmer you will become. Note that pushing your body too hard may cause it to break down.

The best thing that you can do is to set a balance between exercising and dieting. Concentrating only on your workouts may compromise the diet plan that you are planning to follow. You may only end up losing not your excess fat, but your energy. Excessive workouts can actually cause more harm than good. Working out for too long and beyond what your body can take may cause you to suffer from the following:

- Extreme stress, especially because the workouts can disturb your metabolism

- Tiredness, causing the production of more cortisol - Overproduction of this hormone can trigger many health issues including your inability to eliminate your stubborn fats.

- Mental problems – This is usually an effect of your obsession on what you do, as well as your target result.

Now that you are aware of the negative side effects of some instant solutions to weight loss, it is time to learn about what you can do to reach your goal using more natural means. Again, there should be a proper balance between your workout and your chosen diet method. While it's not easy to go natural, it is more advisable than rapid weight loss solutions because it is safer and healthier for you. All you have to do is to start healthier habits and you will eventually adapt to them, making it easier for you to stick 'till the end.

Chapter 3 - Form New Healthy Habits: Appreciate the Process

This section of the book will talk about some of the principles that you can follow, as well as some habits that you can form to finally eliminate your excess belly fats and maintain your slim figure.

Principle #1: Change your mindset

Changing your mindset is the first thing you must do whenever you want to start a diet. It is because your mind - your brain - controls every single thing in your body, so you also have to ensure that you know exactly what you are doing and change your mindset when it comes to dieting, exercising and losing weight.

First of all, think that you need to prioritize your health. This kind of mindset will prevent you from searching for quick weight loss solutions that can only have drastic effect on your health. Not telling yourself the importance of your health will tempt you to try simple and instant methods, instead of exerting an effort to ensure permanent results.

Secondly, you also need to strongly commit to your end goal. Set clear goals; ask yourself why you really want to eliminate your belly fat and achieve a slimmer figure. Is it to look good and feel better about yourself? Is it to improve your health? If you know your exact purpose and goal, you can easily commit to your routines, instead of giving up within just a few tries. Please keep in mind that weight loss cannot be achieved overnight. You have to commit to ensure that all your efforts will produce positive results that can last for a long time.

Third, think of the best weight loss strategies that will work for your case. Look for the most suitable diet and workout plans, and environmental settings for you. Your mindset should also focus on the success of the program. However, you need to make sure that you are also enjoying the process. Do not allow yourself to get too stressed out with the whole process. You have to enjoy the entire process, so you can keep on doing it, instead of giving up.

Principle #2: Changing Old Habits that Destruct your Health

Once you have changed your mindset and committed to stick to a fat burning diet, the next step is to stay away from old habits that may prevent you from reaching your end goal. To form newer and healthier habits, exert an effort to make adjustments. Change your old habits that are destructive to your health including the following:

Excessive Alcohol Consumption

People who don't consume too much alcohol tend to be healthier, and live longer and more productive lives. If you have the habit of drinking alcoholic beverages, especially after a long and stressful day, then it's time to stop. Note that this habit can only increase your blood sugar level and can increase the amount of fats stored in your belly. Most people also drink alcohol at night, which is not good because it is when your body and your metabolism are already at rest. This makes it harder for you to lose the weight that you may have gained from that habit.

Untreated Stress

Modern people receive a lot of stress and pressure from their families, their work, the society where they belong to and even on themselves. Such pressure can trigger anxiety and depression. If left untreated, you may have a hard time finding genuine happiness. Your unhappiness may cause you to be unable to reach your goal. Note that you need to find genuine happiness, since this will serve as an internal, driving force that will motivate you to continue working on your goals.

Real happiness should come from yourself, and you can't expect to get it if you are too stressed. Despite the fact that outward circumstance can also contribute to your happiness, you can actually control your mind and soul to be happy. Learn to live life in a more relaxing manner and learn how to treat stress.

If you find it hard to get rid of stress, then seek professional help. Professionals can help you manage your emotions and your life in a more effective manner, giving you more control over your existence. Once you get rid of stress, you can enjoy a better and happier life, since you can start making more rational decisions.

You may also try seeking for spiritual growth, since many people have already proven its usefulness in overcoming mental issues such as anxiety and stress. Anxiety, depression and stress all contribute to excess fats in your body, especially in your belly, so you should do something to treat or manage them.

Idleness

Being idle is also a habit that you need to change. Keep in mind that you spend long hours being idle, especially during your working days since you sit in front of your computer most of the time. When you have your days off, it is most likely that you spend them on sleeping or doing nothing, so you can give yourself the time to rest. However, remember that idleness is one of the most common contributors to weight gain. Stay active. Move your body from time to time. You don't have to go on rigorous workout routines to keep your body moving. Even doing household chores without using machines is already a huge help in keeping yourself active.

Bad Eating Habits

Some of the bad eating habits that you need to change or stay away from are the following:

- Too much salt or processed and instant food consumption

- Eating or dining out too often – either in fast food chains or fancy restaurants

- Too much sugar and high fat food intake

- Eating even if you are not hungry

- Consuming huge portions of meals

- Eating too often

- Eating less of nutritious foods

- Eating rapidly

- Undereating

- Too much intake of foods rich in starch, gluten and carbs

Develop healthier eating habits that will help you reduce the amount of fat in your body. Remember that you are what you eat, so it is time to pay close attention to what you take in.

Smoking

No explanation needed for this since most, if not all, are already fully aware that smoking can cause your body more harm than good. It's time to quit this habit and focus on living a healthier lifestyle.

Lack of Sleep

A healthy human being should sleep for at least 6 to 8 hours a day. This can give your body enough time to rest. When your body and the organs inside it are resting, you actually charge your energy so that you can start a better day tomorrow. Moreover, adequate sleep will balance your hormones and increase your energy for your workout routines, making it easier for you to reach your weight loss goals.

Not Consuming Enough Water

You need to supply your body with enough water. Instead of taking unhealthy beverages that are rich in sugar and calories, consider drinking pure water. Your body is made up of

75% water, so you need to replenish it from time to time. You need eight glasses of water, around 2 liters, per day. Aside from being useful in hydrating your body, getting enough water also reduces your risk of developing certain ailments like urinary tract infection, colon cancer, urinary stone disease, salivary gland problems and obesity.

Skipping Breakfast

Breakfast is the most important meal of the day. However, many people ignore it because they are busy preparing themselves for work. Ironically, modern people replace their breakfast with a quick visit to a coffee shop and some doughnuts. This is an unhealthy habit that you need to stay away from.

Eating your breakfast can prepare your body for its daily activities. It is important because it can give you the energy that you need to complete all your tasks. You don't have to worry about your body not being able to process and utilize all the foods that you take in in the morning, since it actually does the opposite. Note that you still have a long day ahead, so whatever you consume in the morning will most likely be burned within a few hours.

Waking Up Late

Waking up late will just cause you to rush to do the things that you have to do, thereby lowering your chance of preparing a healthy and hearty breakfast. It may also cause you to miss several opportunities for morning exercises. Try to develop the habit of waking up thirty minutes earlier than your schedule. This will give you some time for yourself. You can use this to meditate, contemplate, prepare a healthy breakfast or exercise.

Principle #3: Appreciating the Process

Instant solutions for weight loss are not recommended due to their negative side effects, so you have to develop the habit of appreciating the process of losing weight no matter how long it is. Be patient, since you will eventually reach your target.

Here are the reasons why you should start appreciating the fat burning process:

- Prepares your body for transformation.

  Note that you can't expect your body to adjust to your new routines and ways of living right away. It needs a warm-up, which means that you have to slowly integrate your new habits, instead of forcing your body to adjust to it right away. If possible, dedicate the first two weeks of your program to preparing your body for positive transformation. It should not only focus on your shape, but also on your body and health as a whole. Giving your body enough time to adjust to the new routines can help it immediately recover from certain issues like laziness, stress and fatigue.

- Prepares your mind and body to focus on the program. This will make it easier for you to sustain the healthy habit for a long time and prevent the risk of giving up.

  Understanding how your brain works is also crucial when implementing new dieting methods. This will make you aware of the potential mistakes that you may commit during the process. You can also train your brain to say no every time you are tempted to go back to your old, unhealthy habits. You will have more control over your mind and body, making it easier for you to reach your target.

Once you have incorporated these three principles in your life, you can start performing belly fat exercises and following the most suitable diet plan for you. Move to the next chapter, so you can discover more effective tips to losing belly fat quickly and sensibly.

Chapter 4 - Sensible Belly Fat Burning Exercises

This chapter has a collection of the most effective belly fat burning exercises that you can do yourself. This will give you plenty of choices when it comes to exercises, but you have to pay close attention to some vital rules before you start. These include the following:

- **Do the exercises on a regular basis** - Be disciplined enough to continue your workout routines, since you can't expect to produce your desired results if you can't follow through. You should also combine exercises with a good dieting program. Eat healthy and nutritious foods, so you can make the most out of your workouts.
- **Avoid pushing yourself too hard** – Note that each person has a different level of strength and flexibility. Some exercises that are very easy for others to do are too difficult for some. Instead of pushing yourself too hard, listen to your body. If you feel like you can't do a certain exercise, then look for another one, which is perfect for you. Practice on what your body can afford to do at first. Sooner or later, your body will be able to adapt to challenging routines.
- **Don't get discouraged if you are still on the stage of familiarizing yourself with the new and healthier lifestyle** – During the first week, it is normal for you to experience muscle pains and tensions. The good news is that you will eventually adapt to the exercises, which means that those pains and tensions are only in the beginning. Don't get discouraged, and continue working out until you reach your goal.

Morning Exercise

Health experts say that it is best to start your day early. Doing so will let you enjoy numerous benefits including the following:

- Enough time to think of yourself - It is beneficial to start your day with clear and happy thoughts and positive mood, so it is advisable to wake up early and use the extra time to do something which is beneficial for you, such as meditation. Some people choose to have a morning prayer. Whatever you do, keep the activity positive by focusing more on yourself.

- Extra time to exercise - Always begin your day with simple, yet useful, exercises. A 15- to 20-minute morning exercise is usually enough, since it can already prepare your body for your daily routines. Spending fifteen to twenty minutes to exercise in the morning is also good for your metabolism.

To start your workouts, here are the most effective ones that you can do even if you are just at home:

On the Bed Workouts

Who said that you need to stand up and wear your gym outfit to exercise? You can actually do your exercises anytime and anywhere. This section of this e-book will provide information on the best exercises that you can do on your bed to get rid of stubborn belly fats.

1. **Stretching**

   Stretching is crucial, especially if you want to prevent muscle injuries. When you sleep, you are giving your muscles the chance to relax. To prevent them from tensing up when you wake up, you should consider doing a few stretches. Here are some steps that you can do to stretch your muscles:

   - Lie down and position your entire body, including your hands and legs, vertically. Stretch out, but avoid stretching too far. Do it slowly, but surely.

   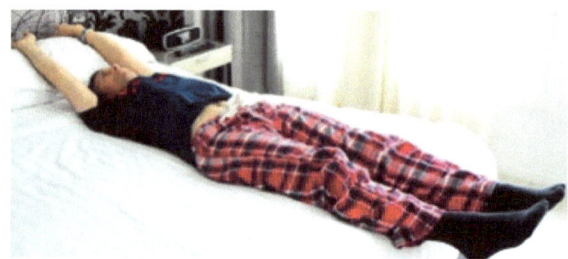

   - After that, move your head and hands. Move your head to the left, then to the right. Stay in each direction for fifteen seconds. Do 3 sets of this specific step.
   - Next, while you are still in the position, take one of your legs to your chest, and keep it for 8 counts (approximately 15 seconds). Do the same on the other leg. Perform 3 sets.

   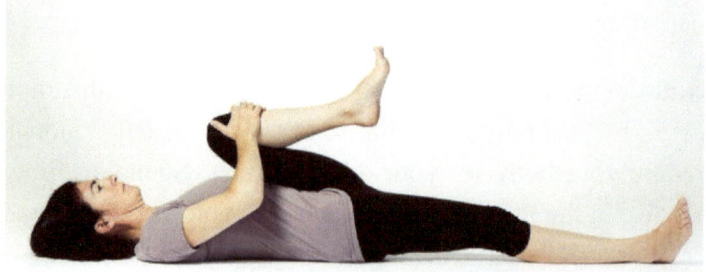

- Take both legs to your chest, then stay in this position for 8 counts. Perform 3 sets.

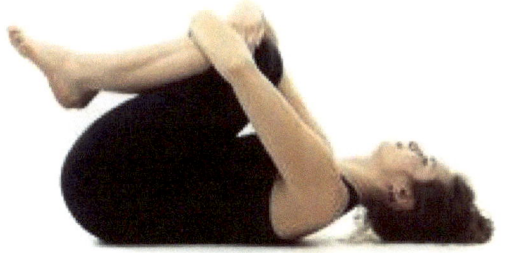

2. Abdominal Twist

After doing a stretching exercise, it would be best to work out your abdominal muscles next. One exercise that targets your abdominal muscles is the abdominal twist. Spread your hands then direct your face on one side while your legs and stomach are on the other side. The goal of this exercise is to shape the sides of your belly so that you can burn fat. Wait for 8 counts before moving on to the other side. Perform 3 sets.

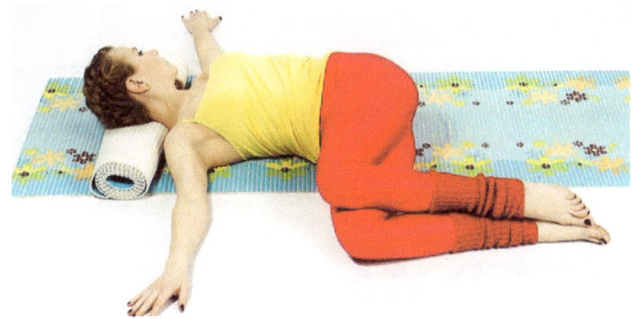

You can also make the abdominal twist even more challenging, if you find it too easy for you. Just place your palms at the back of your head. Bring your legs up, until they form a 45-degree angle. Twist your abs by touching your right elbow to your left knee. You can choose to hold it for 4 counts before moving on to the other side, or move directly to the other side. Perform 4 sets of this exercise.

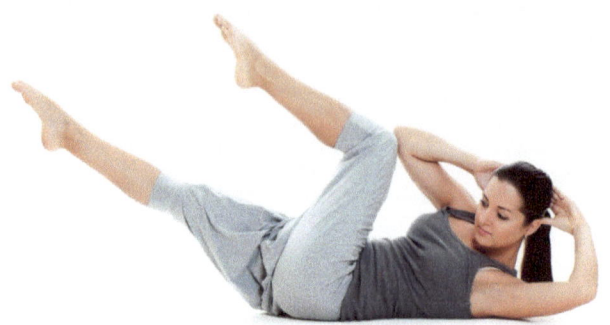

3. Lower Abs Exercise

This posture is so efficient in burning excess fats in your lower abs. Lie down with your palms on the bed first. Take both of your legs up then lift your hip. Stay in this position for 8 counts. Do 4 sets of this exercise.

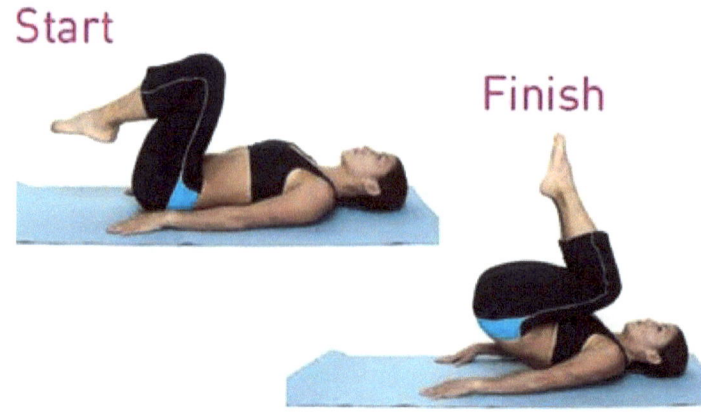

Another lower abs exercise that you can do without having to go to the gym involves lifting your hip while keeping your feet planted on the bed. Lift your body up while you are in that position. Hold this posture for 8 counts and perform at least 4 sets.

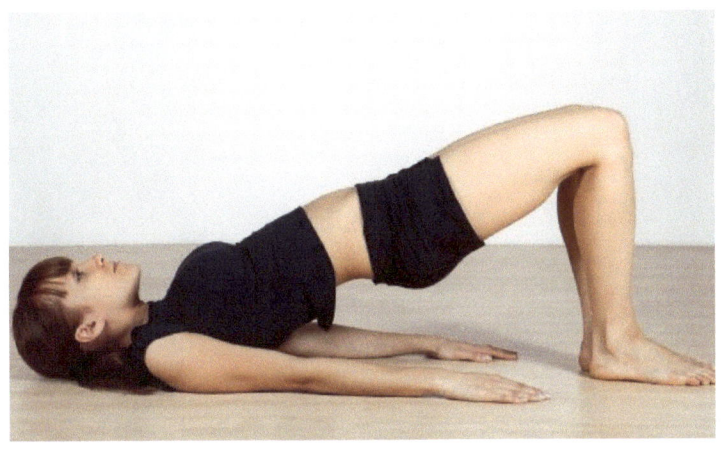

The most difficult lower abs exercise requires more balance than the previous two. Once you get used to the postures above, you can make them more challenging by lifting one foot until it faces the ceiling. Lift your hip then hold that position for 4-8 seconds. To make it easier for you, cross your hands on your chest.

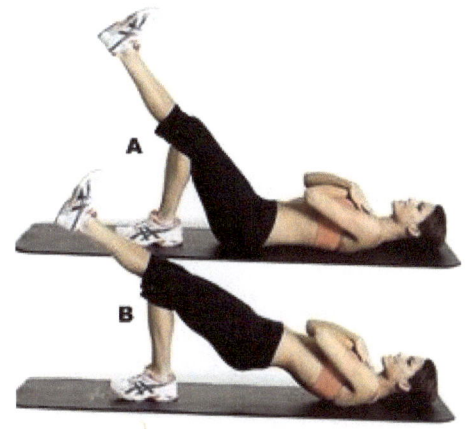

4. Sit ups Challenge

The sit-up is a total abs workout because it targets your abdominal muscles, thereby burning excess fats in your belly. You can actually try several versions of the sit-ups.

The most common one involves placing your hands behind your head, then using them to force yourself to lift your body towards your knees.

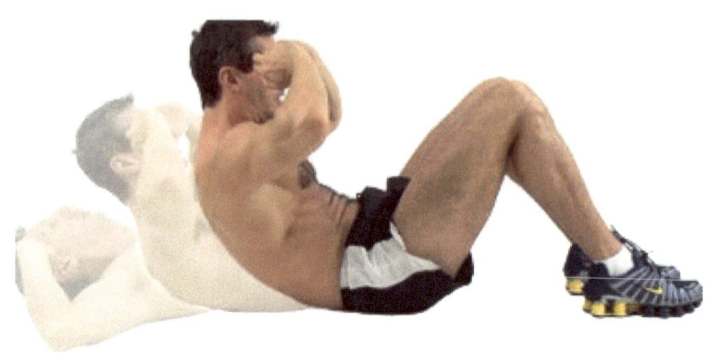

If you find it too difficult to do because you are still a beginner, then you can try the half sit-up version. This is almost the same as the most common version, without lifting your upper body too far.

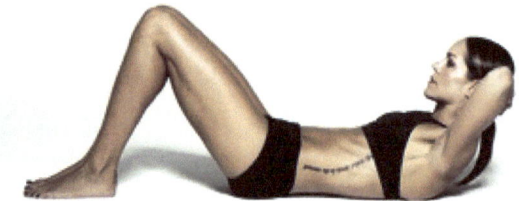

If you are still a beginner, you can do **the half sit-up model** by placing your hands between your thighs or the knees. Your hands will be your driving force to complete the routine.

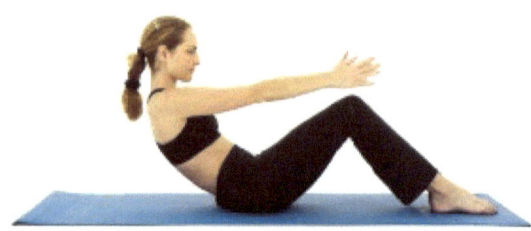

You can do 8 sit-ups. During the last part, hold the last pose for eight counts. Do 4 sets to maximize its effects.

5. Paddling Style

This exercise involves cycling on your bed. Paddling in the air can put a lot of pressure to your lower abdominal muscles and your thighs, thereby allowing you to burn excess fats in the mentioned areas. Raise your two legs to start cycling or paddling in the air. Do it for 8 to 20 times. If you are still a beginner, avoid raising your legs too high since it can cause overexertion and injuries along the process. Allow yourself to get used to the routine first. Once you master this step, you can easily create a 90-degree angle and cycle or paddle in the air without harming yourself.

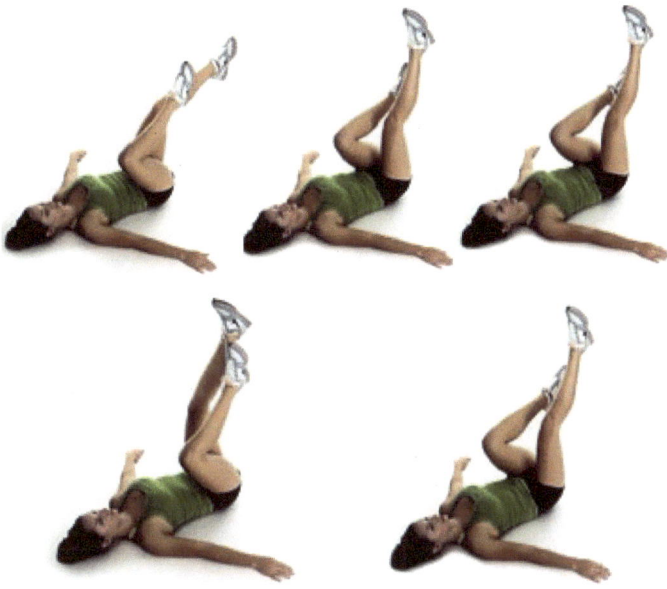

6. Lying upside down belly fat burning

The last part of the "on the bed" workouts is the upside down challenge. It mainly targets your belly fat. To start, turn your body upside down with your hands on your sides. Lift the upper side of your body. This can target your upper ab muscle. Do 8 sets of this step and in the last one, hold the pose for 8 seconds.

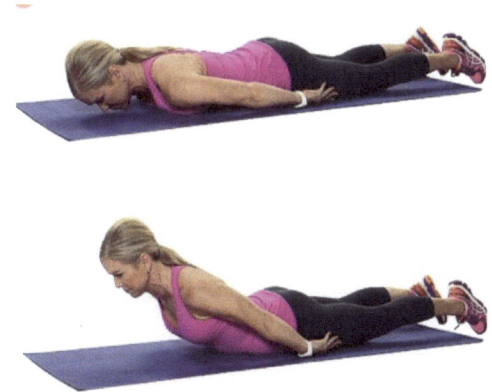

There is also the **scorpion style**, which came from a yoga posture. This can work out your upper and lower abs, since you will be stretching the upper part of your body far to your feet. Place your hands in a comfortable position on the floor, so you can effectively support your upper body. Do this pose for approximately 8 seconds. Breathe slowly and feel your muscles are stretching out. Do 4 sets of this step.

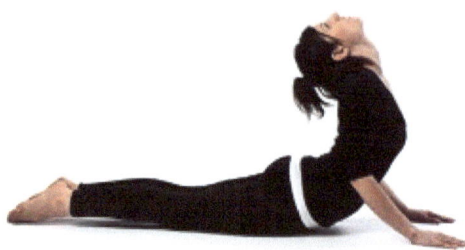

The last one under this category is the **wheel pose**. You can do this routine if you have already gained enough flexibility from your previous workouts. A lot of those who tried this out also say that it works effectively in flattening their belly.

Lie upside down and hold your feet with your hands, until you are forming a wheel. Hold this position for 8 seconds, then relax. Do it again. It is recommended to do 4 sets of this exercise to achieve the best results.

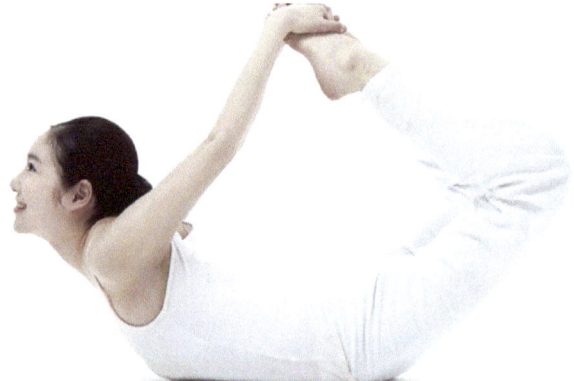

Stomach Pumping for Better Metabolism

In yoga, there is a specific pose or routine, which helps improve your metabolism - stomach pumping. Here is a step by step guide on how to do it:

1. Stand up straight with your hands on your side. Avoid positioning your legs too far from each other. Just leave enough space in between them.
2. Bend a little bit and start pumping your stomach.

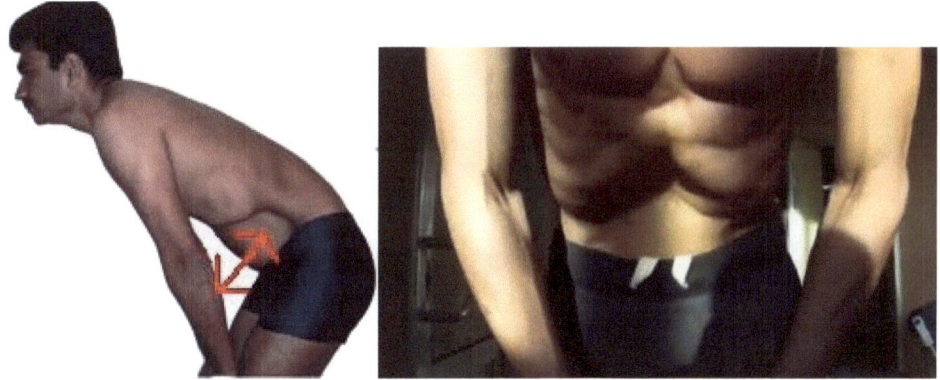

3. Pumping your stomach is also possible even if you are lying down. See the figure below.

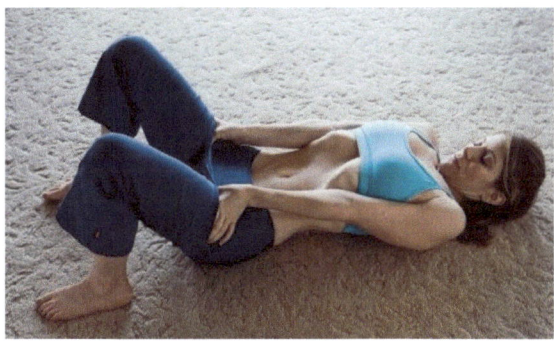

4. Start this routine slowly for 8 times, then go harder in the next 8 reps. Rest then do it again for 4 times.

Office Workout

The good thing about working out is that you can find some workouts that you can do even if you are in your office. If you are working in the office, then it is most likely that you are spending too much time sitting in front of your computer. If you don't move, then there is a great possibility that you will continue to store extra fats in your belly.

The good news is that you can perform a few exercises even if you are at work, thereby preventing your belly from accumulating more fats. You can do some of the exercises mentioned in this section when you are either standing up or sitting in your office chair.

Seated Exercises

Many office workers have extra fats not only in their belly, but also in the lower parts of their bodies like the thighs, bottoms and legs due to the lack of physical movements. The following exercises are designed to help you burn fat in your lower abdomen and the other parts of your lower body.

1. Bowing Exercise

This is probably one of the easiest exercise that you can do when you are sitting in your computer chair. It comes in two types – the half-bowing and the full-bowing exercise.

The **half-bowing exercise** is perfect for you if you want to target the upper part of your belly. Bow one time, hold this position for 4 seconds then sit back. Do this 4 to 8 times during your break time.

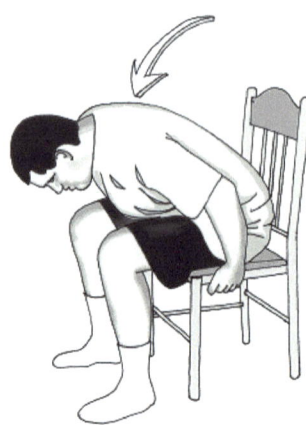

The full-bowing exercise involves bowing forward so that your hands are already touching the ground. This can add more pressure on the upper part of your belly, thereby getting rid of excess fats in the area. Hold this pose for a longer time (preferably 8 seconds). Repeat at least 8 times.

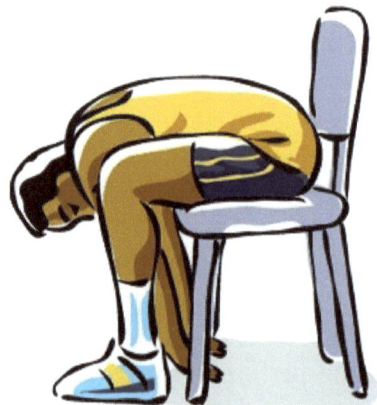

2. Legs up

You can also do a workout in your office that burns excess fats not only in your lower abs, but also in the inner parts of your thighs. Sit properly with your forearms parallel to the ground. After that, lift one of your legs until it forms a 90-degree angle to your upper body. Make sure that the other knee is also bending at a 90-degree angle. Hold this position for 8 seconds.

Next, slowly bring it back to the ground, then repeat the previous steps on the other leg. Do this for 8 to 20 times. Relax your legs afterward.

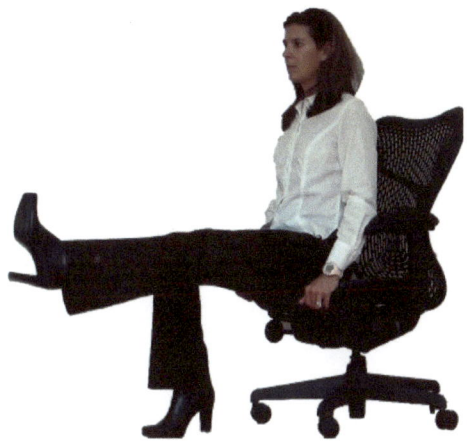

After doing this exercise one leg at a time, you can try a more challenging version, which involves raising both your legs, still forming a 90-degree angle to the upper part of your body. This is more challenging, making it possible for you to burn more fats in your inner thighs and belly. It can also prepare your lower abs for your next exercise. If you add more tension and pressure to your lower abs, then it means that you are effectively burning fat in that area.

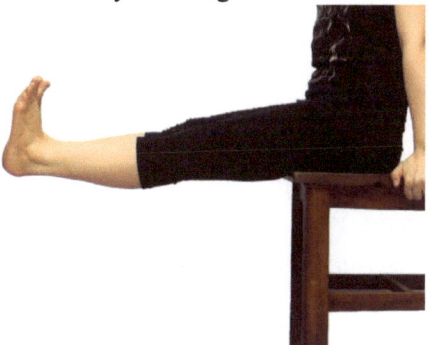

3. Thighs ups and downs

Once you're done with your legs, it's time to target your thighs. The idea is the same, which is to add more pressure and tension to the lower abs so that you can burn fat easier in the area.

Sit down properly with your back against chair. Put your palms under your thighs then raise them slowly. Hold this position for 8 seconds and return to the sitting position. Repeat for 8 to 20 times to maximize its effects.

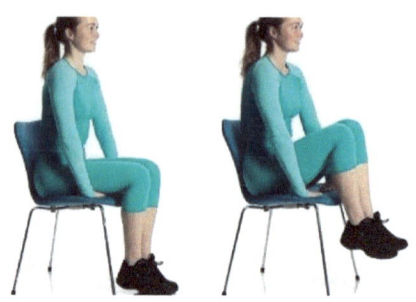

If you want to make it more challenging, lift your bottoms a bit then lean backwards in such a way that you are already placing your back against the chair. Place your hands at the back of the chair then slowly raise your thighs. Stay in this position for 4 to 8 seconds then lower your thighs. Do it for 8 to 20 times.

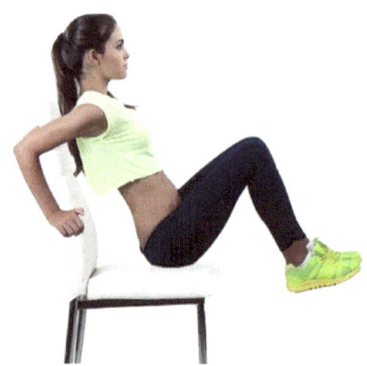

4. Tummy Twist

This exercise targets your abdominal muscles. To work out these muscles even more, make sure to do 20 sets of tummy twist. Sit on your working chair while facing on one side. Place one hand around the back of your chair, then twist your body to the opposite side. This is extremely useful in burning excess fats on the sides of your belly.

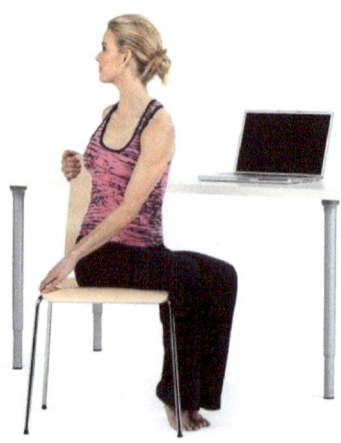

To make it an overall abs and thigh fat burning exercise, raise one of your legs, place your hands behind your shoulders, and let the opposite elbow touch the lifted leg. Do the same on the opposite side. Do 20 sets.

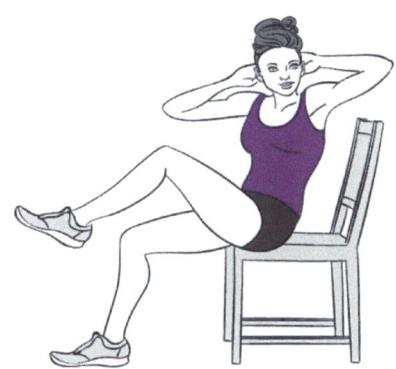

5. Butt Dipping

This exercise is a bit more difficult and challenging than the other exercises that were already mentioned in this chapter, so avoid forcing yourself to do it if you are still not used to the routine.

Master this exercise slowly, but surely. It targets your arms, abs, thighs and legs, which means that it is a full workout routine that you can do even if you are sitting.

Sit on the tip of the chair. Make sure to position your hands on the chair comfortably, so you can use them to support your weight later on. Move halfway off the chair, moving towards the floor. Dip your bottoms towards the floor, but make sure that they don't touch the ground.

Move up again, then return to your original sitting position. Do this movement several times, based on how much reps you can afford to do.

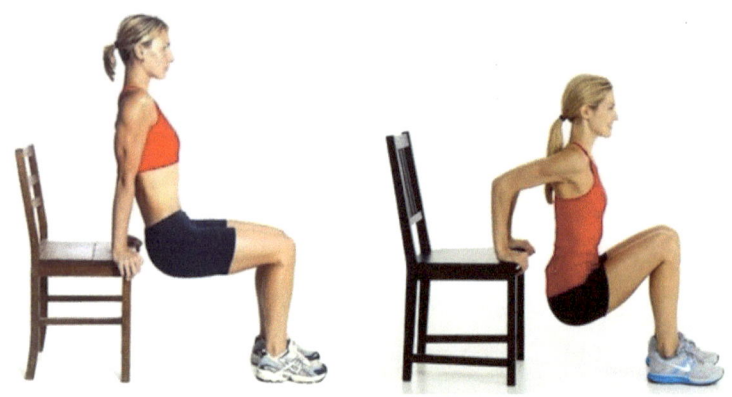

Familiarize yourself with the seated exercises mentioned in this chapter, so you can start doing them even if you are in your office. The main goal of these exercises is to ensure that you stay active even if you are in your workplace. Aside from the mentioned exercises, simple routines, like climbing the stairs in the office, are already enough to keep you moving and help you take full control of your weight.

Stay-at-home Workouts

The next exercises are for those who often stay at home.

On the Sofa Workouts

You can do various things while sitting in your sofa - from leg paddling to butt dipping. Instead of watching TV, do some workouts. You can also perform the on the bed and the seated workouts mentioned earlier while you are in your sofa.

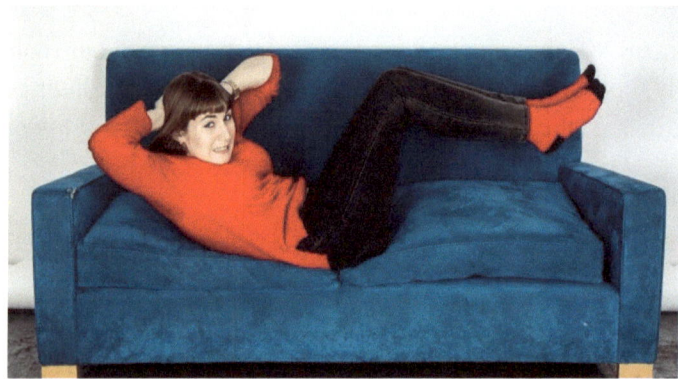

You can also do **push-ups** while on the sofa. The first one is to use the sofa to support your leg, so that you can easily do several reps of push-ups.

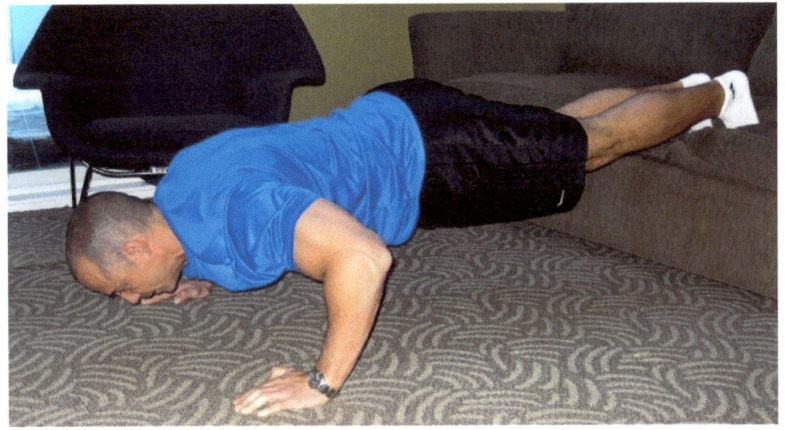

If you find the previous version too difficult for you, then use the arm of your sofa. Just put your hands on the arm of the sofa and do normal push-ups.

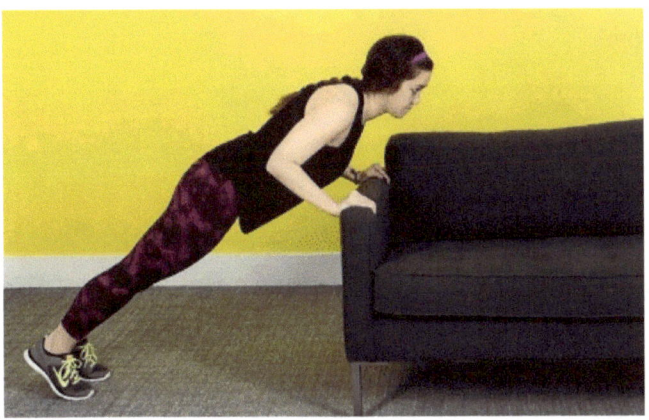

The good thing about push-up is that it is a full body exercise, which means that aside from targeting your abdominal area, you are also working out the other parts of your body.

Making Use of the Stairs

You can use the stairs to perform one popular exercise called **step-ups**. If you don't have any stairs at home, then you can use a box capable of supporting your legs. Climb up and down the box or stair for several times. For a beginner, doing 30 to 50 sets is usually enough. Once you get used to the routine, you can make it more challenging by trying to complete up to 200 sets.

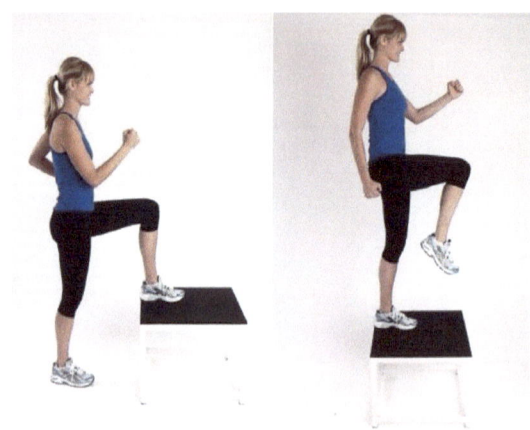

You can also make this exercise more challenging with a **side movement**. This means that instead of climbing up and down while facing the box or stairs in front of you, place the box on your side, or stand beside the stairs. You can then start stepping up and down while in this position.

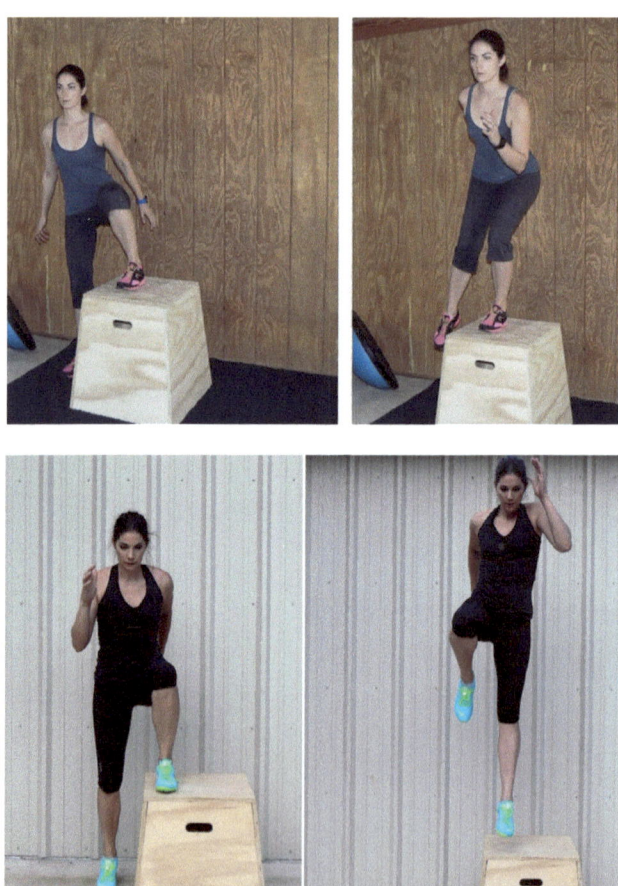

One benefit of step ups is that they target the lower part of your body, starting on your stomach and belly. You can also make use of a solid chair for this. Just make sure that it is strong enough to support your weight and the activity.

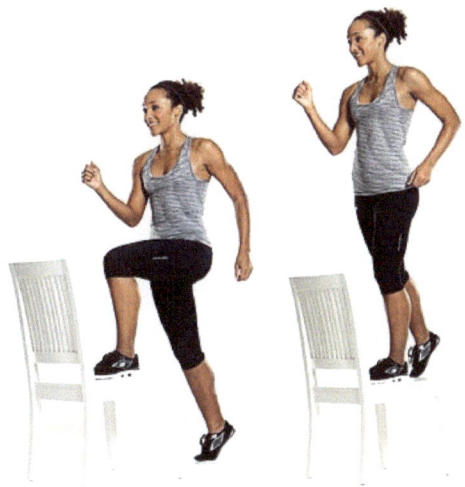

If you want it to become more challenging, then you can jump, instead of just moving up and down normally on the stairs, box or chair.

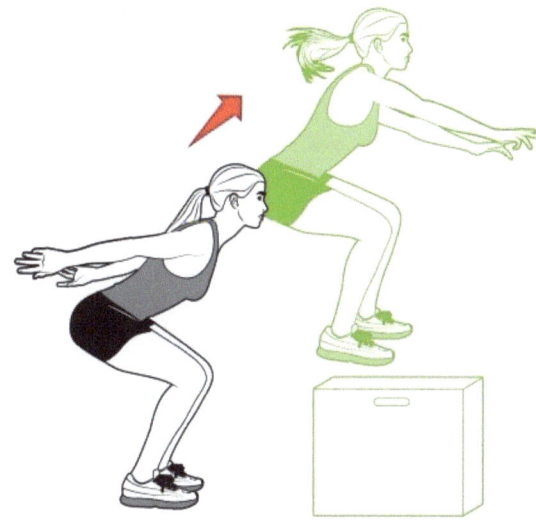

This variation is more effective in burning excess fats since it requires you to use more energy.

Burpees

Squat then kick your feet back. Follow this step with a push-up then return to your squatting position. The last step is to stand up and jump in the air as high as possible.

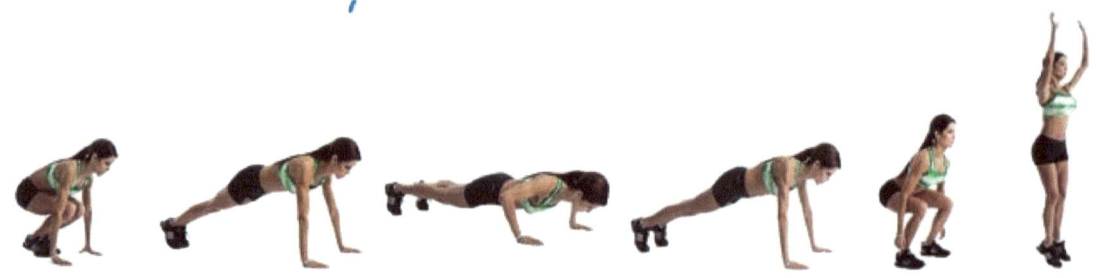

If you are still a beginner, you can do only 8 sets because this routine is already enough to make you feel worn out. Once you gain more experience on this routine, you can start increasing the number of sets that you can perform. However, avoid pushing yourself too hard. A maximum of 20 burpees is usually enough.

On-Screen Tutorial of your Favorite Exercises

You can also play workout videos at home. Follow the instructions on the video, and make sure to do the activity on a regular basis, preferably two or three times per week. If you have enough time to do it every day, then that would be even better. The good thing about working out by viewing workout videos is that you'll also see lean and healthy people on screen. This will further motivate you to continue your exercises. You can also ask someone close to you to work out with you to make the routine more enjoyable.

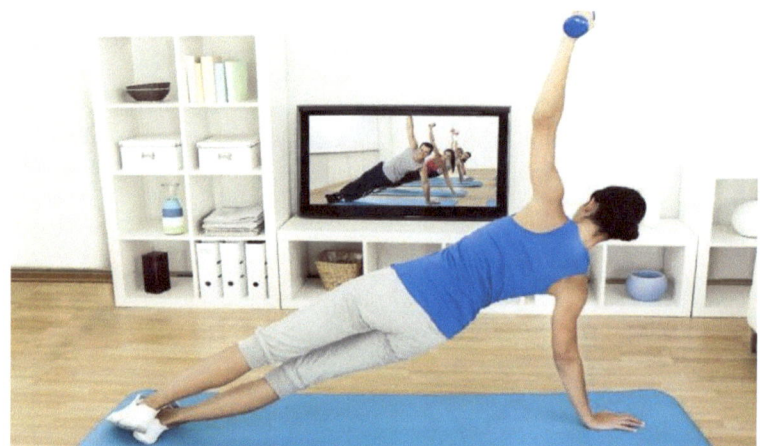

Before-you-sleep Exercises

It is also important to do before bed exercises. However, avoid doing heavy workouts at night because you may have a hard time sleeping once your energy levels go up due to the exercise. Light exercises are usually enough. The goal of these exercises is to keep your metabolism working even when you are already asleep. This will allow your digestive system to digest and process the foods you eat well, making it easier for you to lose weight.

Wall Sit

Place your body against the wall and move downward as if you were sitting on a chair. Hold for 4 to 8 seconds. Do this position for 20 to 40 times.

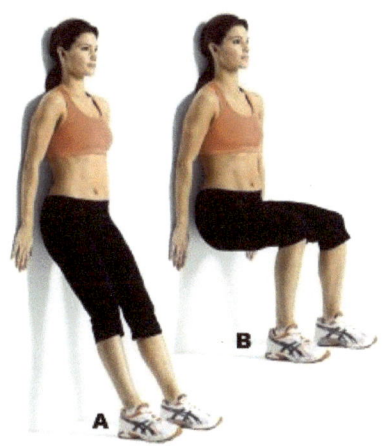

Planks

Planks come in different variations. You can choose from the forearm plank, side plank, standard plank, and reverse plank. Choose one, which you feel comfortable to do. As you gain more experience in this routine, you can perform more challenging variations.

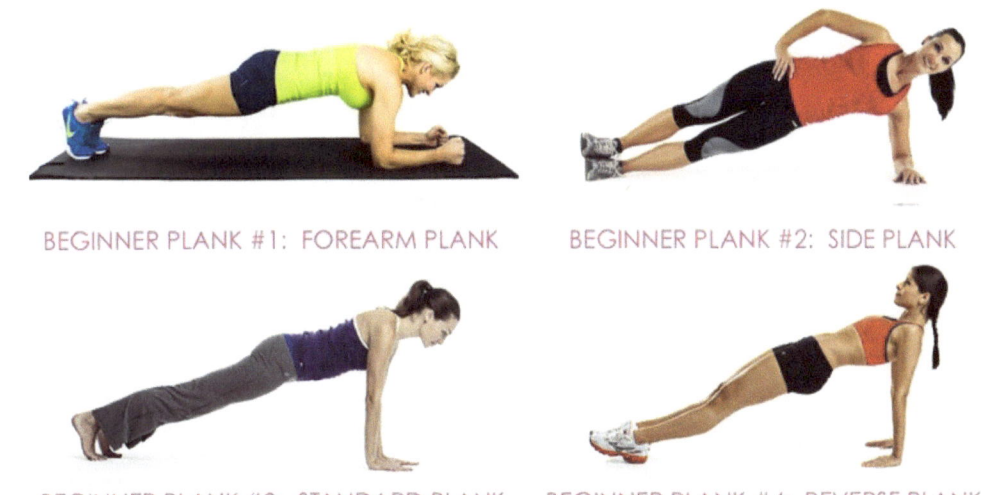

BEGINNER PLANK #1: FOREARM PLANK   BEGINNER PLANK #2: SIDE PLANK

BEGINNER PLANK #3: STANDARD PLANK   BEGINNER PLANK #4: REVERSE PLANK

You can also modify this exercise by raising one of your legs or hands.

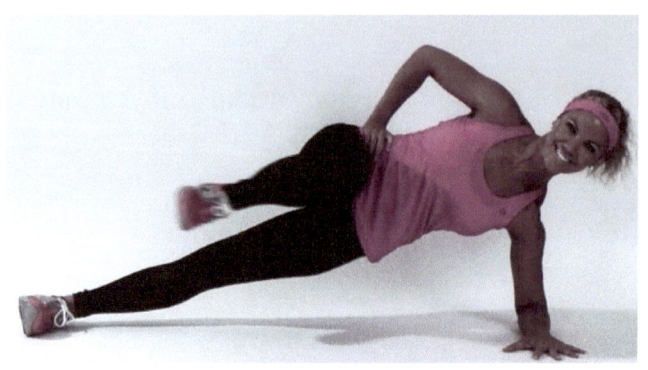

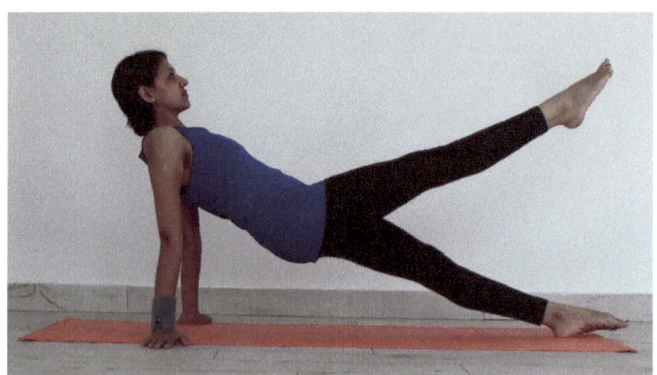

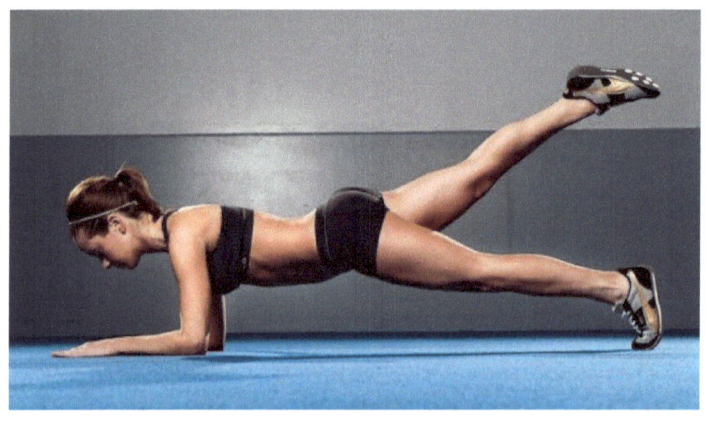

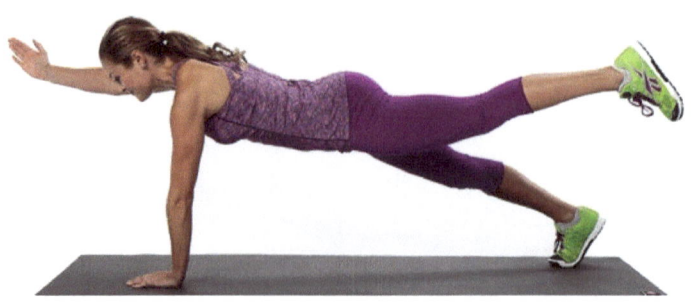

Crunches

You can do crunches both at night and in the morning. Aside from being easier to do than other workouts, crunches are also effective in shaping your abs.

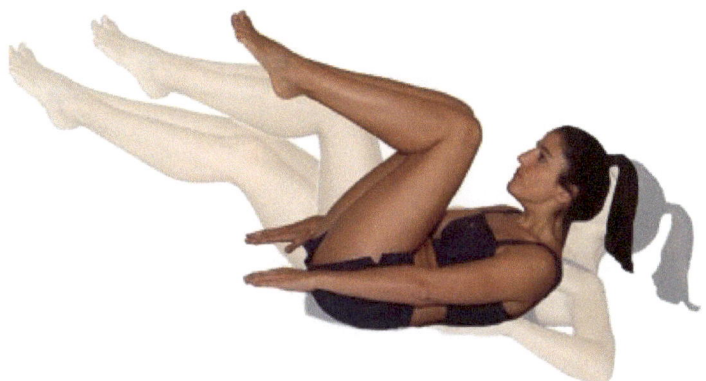

If you want to shape both your upper and lower abs, then consider using your hands and upper body when performing the exercise. Twisting your body during the process also works in burning excess fats on the sides of your belly.

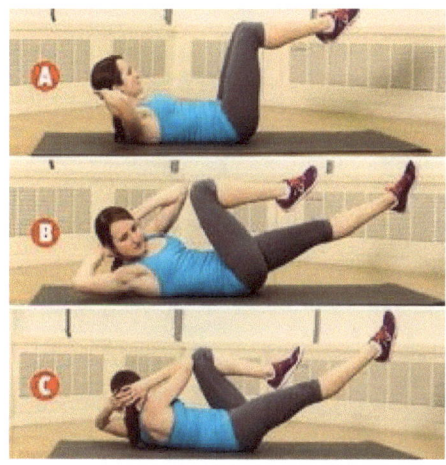

Feet on the wall exercises

First, lie down on the floor and put both your feet on the wall. It is okay to start pumping your stomach for 4 sets before moving to the next step.

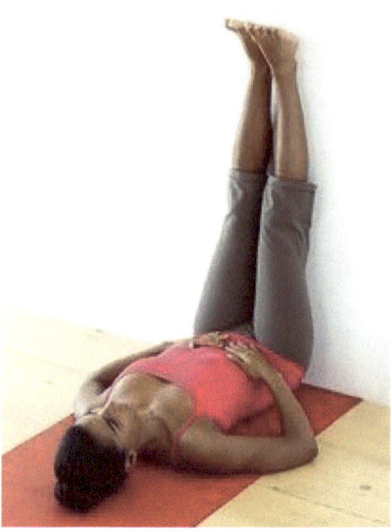

Next, raise one hand after another and use them to force your upper body up. This step is really helpful in reducing fat. Once you feel tired, take a rest. Repeat as necessary (depending on the physical strength of your body).

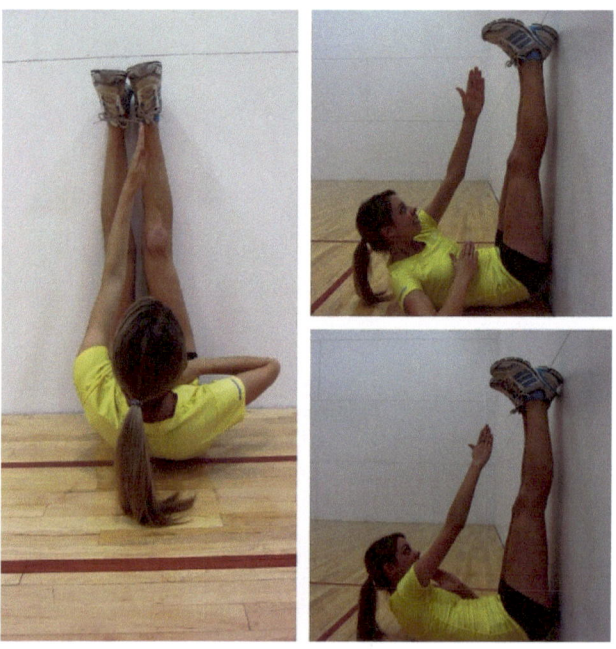

Another variation of feet on the wall exercise is to lift your hip. Bend your knee and press your feet against the wall first, then simply lift your pelvis. Do it 8 times.

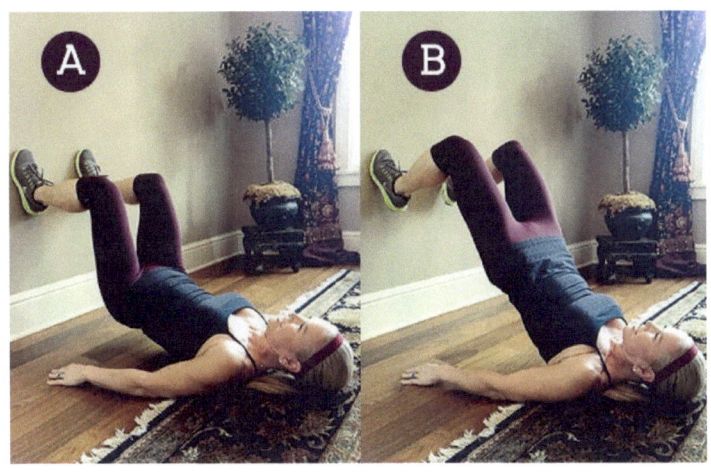

Stability Ball Abs Exercises

One great advantage of using a stability ball to exercise is that it reduces the risk of muscle pains. Moreover, it can help you achieve more balance while also supporting your weight well.

Basically, you can do all of the ab exercises mentioned earlier with the help of the stability ball. All you need to do is to adjust your posture, so that you can effectively use the ball.

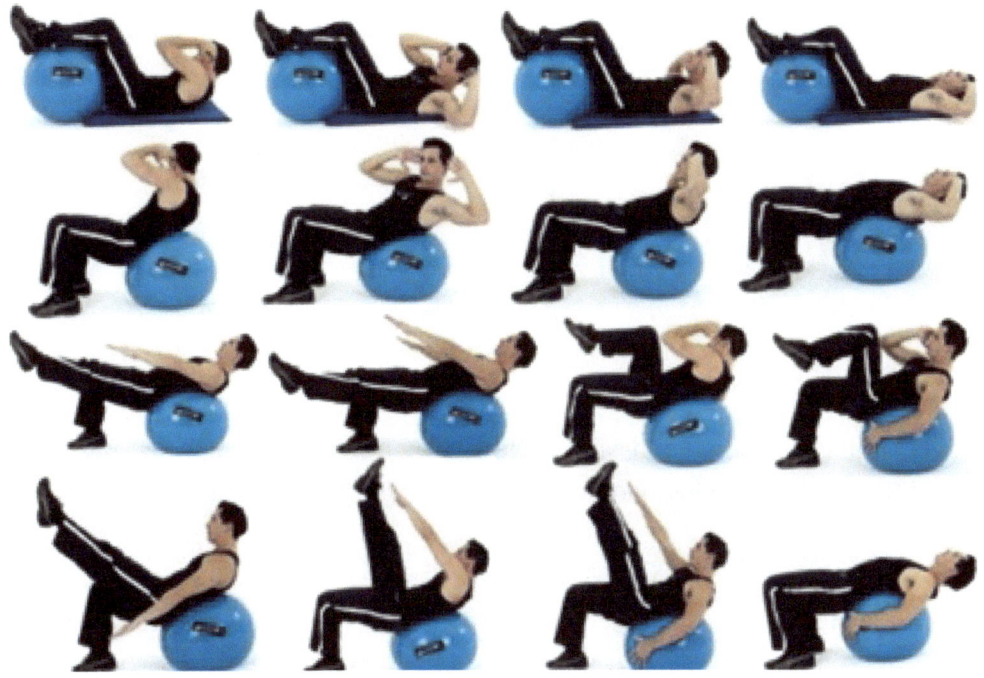

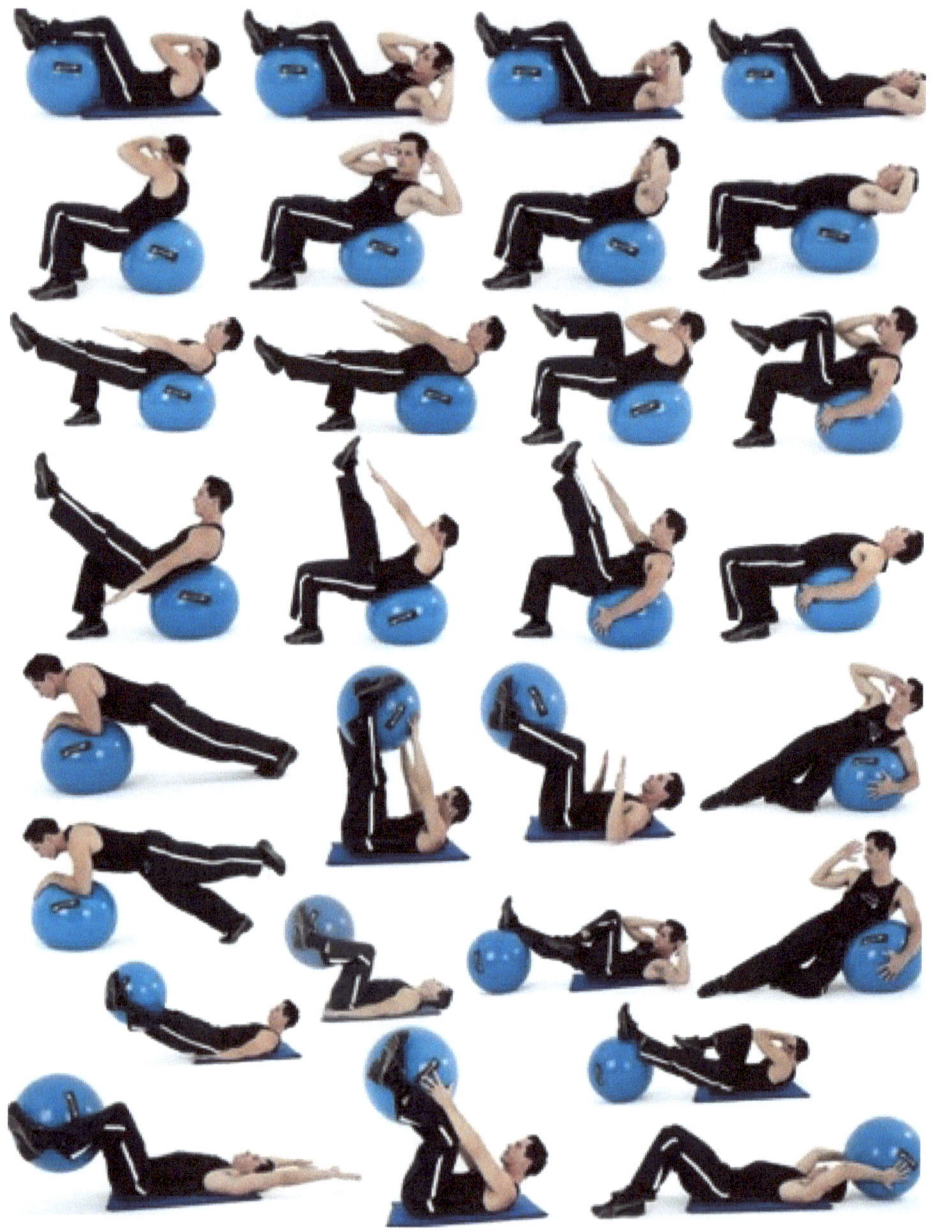

Exercising with the stability ball is also perfect for before-bed exercises because you don't need to push yourself too hard to handle certain steps and positions.

Weekend exercises

You can still exercise even during the weekends. If you want to add more fun and excitement to your workout, especially during the weekends when you are supposed to rest, you can do the following suggestions:

Outdoor Exercises

Take your exercise mat outdoors. You can go to the nearest park or beach to workout. A morning exercise in your backyard is also a great idea. The goal is to make your exercise more fun and exciting by doing it outdoors. You can also find a companion to make it even more exciting.

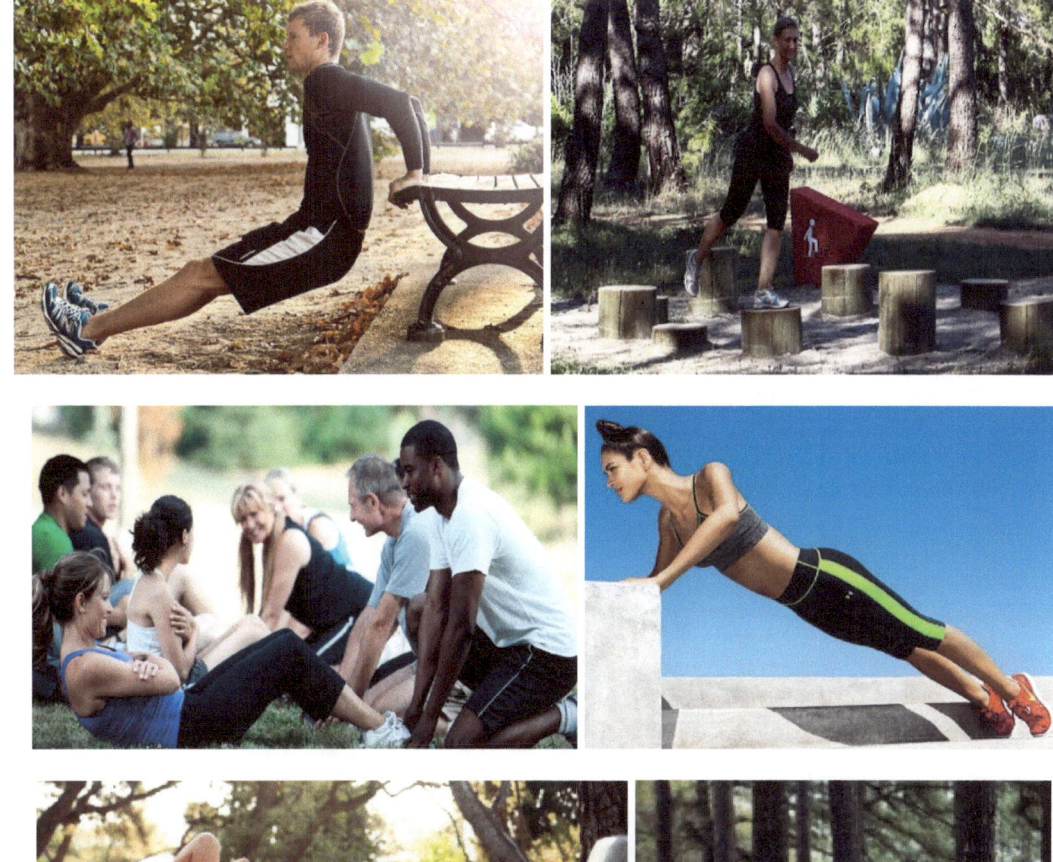

Couple Exercises

Aside from exercising outdoors, you can also do those workouts that involve two people. You can do these routines with your partner, or a close friend. You can even do it with your kid. This can make the entire routine more exciting since you are doing it with a buddy. See the following figures to give you an idea about the exercises that you can do with a partner.

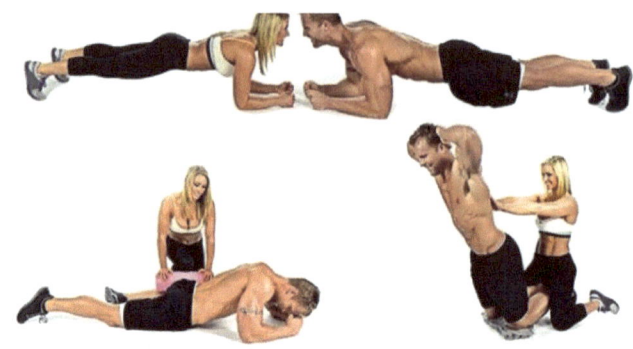

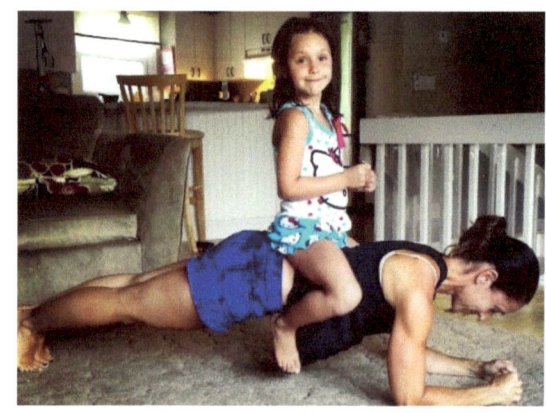

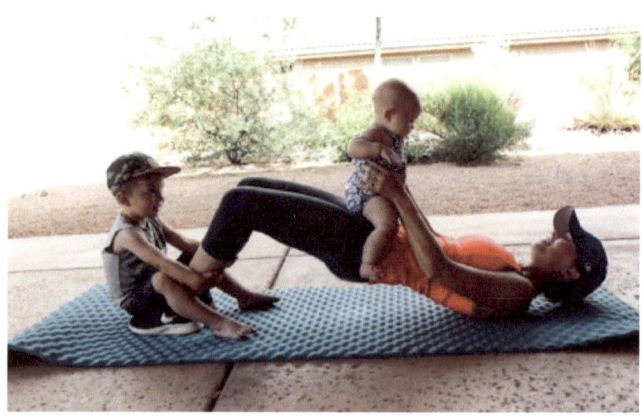

Chapter 5 - Belly Fat Reduction Diet Plans

Now that you are aware of the different exercises that are effective in getting rid of belly fat, it is time to look for the best diet plan for you. As what have been mentioned earlier, exercising is not enough. You need to pair it with the right diet. Before you start your new diet plan, you have to keep in mind that your digestive system also needs to adjust to the new routines. You often need around 14 days to ingest the habits into your system.

With that in mind, here is a 2-week diet plan that will help you jumpstart your new habits and make the process of sticking to them easier. Once you get used to them, you can add some modifications based on your needs and preferences.

2-Week-Diet-Plan to Kick Off New Habits

Day	Morning Habits	Day Time Habits	Before Sleeping Habits
1	- Wake up earlier than usual - Do 15 minutes of morning exercises - Eat fruits for breakfast - Eat cranberries and peanuts for snack at around 10am.	- Take your lunch even before you feel too hungry. - Spend around fifteen minutes doing workouts either in your office or at home after lunch. - Start integrating foods rich in fiber into your diet and reduce your carb intake.	- Eat your dinner before 7pm. - Your dinner should consist of foods rich in protein such as boiled eggs or fat-free meat. - Spend around 15 minutes doing mild exercises before sleeping.
2	- Wake up earlier than usual - Jog for 30 minutes. - Eat sugar-free pancake with honey for breakfast - Snack on cashew at around 10 a.m.	- Have lunch before you feel too hungry and finish it before you feel satiated - Do 15-minute exercises whether you are at home or in the office. - Avoid dining at cafeterias or restaurants. Prepare your own foods, if possible, so you can stay away from foods that are rich in saturated fat and MSG.	- Have dinner before 7 p.m. - Take a small portion of vegetable salad plus steamed chicken with herbs - Do a 15-minute exercise before you sleep.
3	- Wake up earlier than	- Your lunch should	- Eat salmon salad with

	usual - Do a 20-minute morning exercise - Get your dose of carbs from boiled corn. - Drink a glass of sugar-free juice taken from your favorite fruits or vegetables - Snack on apple and 10 almonds at 10am.	consist of the following: 1 banana, 2 hard-boiled eggs, and small portion of boiled veggie with herbs. - Spend 15 minutes for your workout.	spinach, tomatoes, asparagus, and balsamic vinegar for dinner. - Do your 15-minute exercise - Avoid eating after 7 p.m. because you have no physical activities at night. This will prevent you from having stubborn belly fat.
4	- Start your day earlier. Wake up at 6am at the latest. - Spend around 10 minutes to meditate. Focus on your breathing and on your intentions. This will allow you to relax before you start your day. - Do your 15-minute morning exercise. - Eat a healthy and hearty breakfast composed of the following: low-fat yogurt smoothie with frozen fruits - Snack on a bowl of oatmeal with fruits or honey	- Have a turkey sandwich with whole-grain bread for lunch - Work out for fifteen to twenty minutes whether you are at home or in the office.	- Have meatballs with tomato sauce for dinner - Do a 20-minute exercise before you sleep
5	- Do a 30 minute morning exercise - Eat your breakfast – scrambled egg from 1 whole egg and 2 egg whites and a small portion of vegetable smoothie.	- Eat something cooked with air fryer for lunch. Add a half of medium-sized baked potato so you can get your required dose of carb. - Work out by climbing the stairs.	- Your dinner should be composed of the following: lean meat steak plus the leftover potato from your lunch. - Do a 20-minute exercise before you

	- Stay away from starchy foods from this day forward.		sleep.
6	- Go cycling for 20 minutes. - Have roasted tuna for your breakfast and a cup of berries for snack.	- Have shrimp salad with vegetable and olive oil for lunch. - Take a walk for around 10-15 minutes.	- Take ricotta with lentils and broth for dinner. - Spend around 20 minutes doing mild exercises before sleeping. -
7	- Do a 10-minute exercise. - Eat an egg sandwich with cucumber - For your snack, one big orange plus a stick string would do. - Start the habit of defecating every morning (before 9 a.m.). This indicates that you have a good metabolism.	- Your lunch should consist of a veggie soup with chicken broth. - Work out by climbing the stairs	- For your dinner, eat one portion of turkey breast and mashed potatoes. - Start the habit of reading books about losing belly fat. You can also watch videos of those who successfully reduced significant amounts of weight, especially in the belly on YouTube. Use this as your motivation to continue. - Rest. You are free to let go of your exercise routine tonight.
8	- Exercise at the nearest park. This is a good thing, since you will be doing the routine outdoors, making it more interesting. - Take a cup of oatmeal with berries for breakfast - Snack on a cup of frozen yogurt and cucumber	- Your lunch should consist of steamed chicken with avocado dip - Exercise for 20 to 30 minutes.	- Prepare fish tacos with onion and cabbage salsa for dinner - Exercise with the help of your favorite abs aerobic video - Try to encourage your loved ones to start dieting, as well. This will let you develop the habits with someone who can

			motivate you.
9	- Wake up earlier than the previous days. - Contemplate or meditate for at least 15 minutes - Review your goals and see the progress you have made so far. - Do a simple on the bed exercise for 10 minutes. - Have a simple breakfast composed of fresh veggies with almond sauce - Prepare a healthy juice for snack	- Prepare white fish filet with steamed broccoli and sweet potatoes for lunch - Go to the nearest park after work to exercise - Eat a small portion of food rich in carb to get a good supply of energy.	- Have grilled turkey breast with asparagus for dinner. - Do simple against the wall exercise for around 15 minutes.
10	- Start early with a 5-minute prayer or meditation - Spend 20 minutes working out in your backyard or balcony. - Eat your breakfast composed of low-fat Greek yogurt with honey and berries. - Snack on a bar of homemade protein bar (almond, cashews, or peanut bars).	- Bake salmon and mushrooms with herbs, serve with a cup of brown rice and raw vegetables, and eat it for lunch - Do 15-30 minutes daytime workouts - Explore your surroundings and find out if there is something that you can do to make your workouts even more challenging or interesting.	- Prepare sardine bruschetta toast with cucumber and tomato for dinner. - Do sofa exercises for 20 minutes before you sleep. - While lying on your bed, check out your 10-day abs diet plan. Review your progress so far, so you will know what to improve and what to preserve in your current habits.
11	- Do a 20-minute morning exercise. Your exercise should focus on your lower abs and thighs. - Eat a small portion of roasted chicken breast with green	- Eat chicken breast with green beans and half-portion of white rice for lunch. - Do a 20-minute daytime workout - Climb up and down the stairs for your workout.	- Have tuna and lettuce salad for dinner. Serve it with mashed or baked potatoes. - Do a 20-minute before bed exercise. - If you feel like your muscles are worn out,

	beans for breakfast. - Walk to the office and take public transportation to increase your physical movements.		then rest assured that it signifies that your exercises are effectively burning fats.
12	- Do a 20-minute morning exercise. Focus on your upper abs and thighs. - Eat your breakfast composed of one portion of homemade fruits or raisin muffin (with less sugar) - Walk to the office and take public transportation or cycle to work.	- Eat chicken or turkey quesadillas with chopped pineapple and celery for lunch - Take a walk after work. - Be part of a diet group and meet people with the same interest as you. If you cannot find one, form one with your closest friends or your family members/relatives. Your group will serve as a great source of motivation.	- Prepare a huge portion of garden salad with lean meat steak. - Burn extra fat by doing the ab twist for around 20 minutes
13	- Do a 20-minute morning exercise. Do more sit-ups and step-ups. Jump to burn more fats. - Take a glass of skimmed milk and egg sandwich with fresh veggies for breakfast	- Have white fish fillet with boiled broccoli and sweet potatoes for lunch. - Work out for thirty minutes. - Make it a habit to reduce the amount of salt and sugar that you take in for lunch and dinner.	-Eat 6 crackers, a cup of low-fat cottage cheese and half-ounce of mixed nuts for dinner. - Do a regular 15-minute exercise before sleeping.
14	- Wake up early and have 1 hardboiled egg with green salad and olive oil for breakfast. - Celebrate your 14th day of abs diet by going to a place that can make your workout experience	- Take the leftover green salad and top it with three slices of baked turkey for lunch. - Because you were able to burn a lot of fats in the morning, you can take a rest. Have a short nap. - Take a handful of	- Prepare sauté shrimp with kale and paprika. Serve with one boiled corn. - Review your 2-week effort and reward yourself for minor and major accomplishments. - Have a weighing

more fun and interesting. Walk to the nearest forest or cycle with your partner. - Drink plenty of water. - Always start your day with a glass of warm or room temperature water. This can speed up your metabolism.	cashews or almond for snack.	scale beside your bed, so you can continue to monitor your weight. Take pictures of yourself, especially around the belly area, every two weeks, so you can clearly see your progress.

Congratulations! You have just finished your 2-week diet plan. The only thing left for you to do is to continue sticking to the new and healthy habits that you have developed. Avoid pushing yourself too hard, however. Note that it is alright to take a break from time to time. For instance, you can take a rest for a day after doing 4 days of routine exercises.

Continuing the Healthy Habits

Incorporate the following things in your diet plan, so you can stick to your new and healthy habits for a long time.

1. Always wake up early in the morning, so you can have enough time for yourself. You can use it to meditate or do additional workouts in the morning. Waking up early can also give you enough time to prepare a healthy breakfast and lunch.
2. Consume one or two glasses of water right after waking up in the morning. This will keep you hydrated and jumpstart your metabolism.
3. The best snacks that you can take when you are still on the dieting phase are a handful of cashews, peanuts and almonds.
4. Have sugar-free fresh juice or smoothies. Add low-fat yogurt or skimmed milk to your smoothies, and natural honey to enhance flavor.
5. Take a break from exercise every once in a while, preferably every 4-5 days. However, you still need to watch out your food intake during your break.
6. Stay away from starch, and take a small portion of carb-rich foods for lunch and dinner.
7. Ask someone close to you to do the routines together. This way, both of you can motivate each other. You can also take part in groups with the same interest as you.

8. Always cook your own meal. Use healthy oils and avoid MSG. Avoid canned, instant and processed foods and eat in moderation.

Chapter 6 - Maintaining your Flat Belly

Now that you have developed new and healthy habits, it is time to learn how you can maintain them. Remember that dieting is a continuous process. While others can accomplish their goals within just a short of time, others spend more time before seeing their desired results. Respect your own process because each person is different, which also makes his ability to adjust to the program different. With discipline and patience, you can lose your belly fats within three months.

Tips in Maintaining your Flat Stomach

1. Remember the objectives of your diet plan. Review the importance of physical and mental readiness when embracing a healthier lifestyle. If you are determined enough, you won't give up until you reach your desired results.
2. You have to commit to the plan. Set goals and put them in writing. Post your written goals in a place where you can see them every day. This will remind you of your goal, thereby ensuring that you will continue to commit to the program.
3. Temptations are everywhere. There are times when you will be tempted to eat foods that are prohibited in the program like chips, pizza, spaghetti and fatty and starchy foods. Develop the willpower and discipline to avoid such temptations. Make it a habit to cook your own versions of the unhealthy foods that you are craving for, so you can add healthier ingredients. For instance, you can make a pizza from cheesy spinach and ground meat or tuna filet with its crust from oatmeal or whole grains.
4. Pay close attention to your environment. Make sure that it is conducive to your diet plan and your workout routines to prevent you from going back to your unhealthy habits.
5. Eat in a restaurant, which serves fresh and healthy ingredients. This is important if you plan to dine out. Be specific when you are already ordering. Ask the waiter if there are healthier versions to the foods that they regularly offer.
6. Remind yourself of your goal through visualization. This is possible by posting a picture of a slim figure in your wall to remind you of what you want to become in the future. This will inspire you to continue dieting and working out until you reach your goal.
7. Make sure that your entire family is involved. Introduce them to the new and healthy habits that you are currently following, so everyone in your household will gain all the benefits of your chosen program.
8. Join a community with the same values and habits as yours. Get a gym membership, so you can meet other people with the same struggle as yours. You can listen to their belly fat reduction stories, learn from their experiences and be inspired.

The choice is in your hands. If you have gone far, avoid quitting since it will only result to you going back to your old and unhealthy routines. Continue with the plan and be ready to face the newer, healthier and slimmer you.

Conclusion

Congratulations! You have just finished the entire book. Now, it's time to choose the best fat burning exercises that are suitable for you. Also, make it a point to adapt healthier diet plans by incorporating them to some of your favorite healthy menus. Create meals on a personal level – that is, you have to prepare them based on your preferences. This will make it easier for you to follow the plan.

Just make sure that you are fully ready for the entire program. Prepare yourself physically and emotionally, so you can embrace a healthier lifestyle and exert an effort to make it work. Stay committed and avoid giving up in the middle of the journey. You can't sustain the results of the program if you instantly quit. You also need to keep in mind that it is a life-long process that you need to appreciate.

You also need to celebrate your achievements – even if you just reduced a small amount of weight. You will most likely stick to the program if you reward yourself for all the accomplishments that you've made.

Happy exercising and following the plans.

JO HANSEN

Check Out Other Books

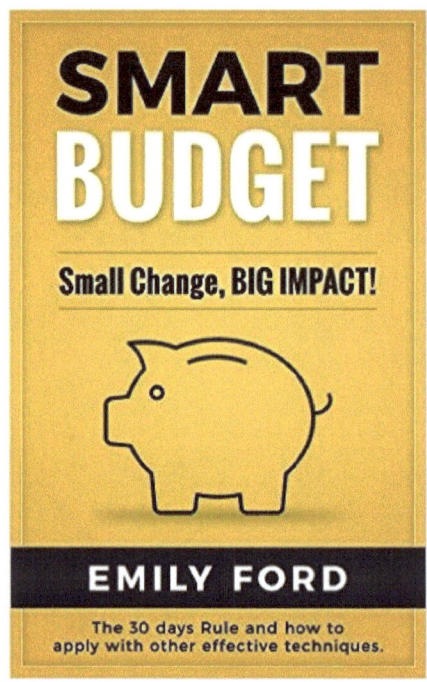

Emily Ford, Author of Smart Budget, shares her real life experiences on how she saved more than $8000 within 30 days! She will also show you how she managed to accumulate more than $1825 with very little effort within a span of 13 months and how you can grow this amount of money to more than $9000 in 5 years.

Many do not understand the importance of managing their finances and to save for the future. They tend to splurge unnecessarily, only to regret once they start struggling to support their own needs and the needs of their family.

It's time to break free from the habit of splurging your hard-earned money on things that don't really matter. Learn how to take control of your finances.

Build your wealth using proven money saving techniques to enjoy a brighter future, live a less stressful life, provide for your loved ones and enjoy your retirement.

FIND THIS BOOK ON AMAZON

https://amazon.com/dp/B01GN8PZQ6